How To Box
Training For Boxing

By
Kerry Pharr

Contact Kerry Pharr
Email: kwpharr@gmail.com
Web-site: www.ProBoxingTrainer.com

Other Titles by Kerry Pharr

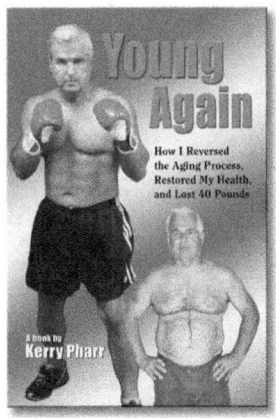

Approaching 60, Kerry Pharr, who considered himself a picture of health during the prime of his life, now viewed himself as "old, fat and sick." Not liking the way he felt and what he was seeing in the mirror. Pharr began to eat a living foods, alkaline, diet that he combined with a pro boxer's conditioning program.

The accidental result was a diet and exercise program that reversed the aging process, restored his health, and helped him lose 40 pounds.

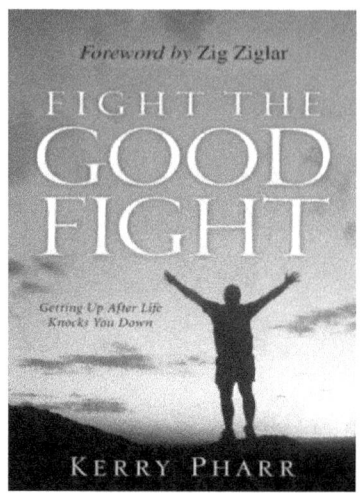

In his book Fight The Good Fight Kerry Pharr tells many stories from the boxing world, including rubbing shoulders with champions Muhammad Ali, John Tate, Sugar Ray Leonard, and Tommy Hearns. He also describes how he contemplated suicide after losing his first wife Diane to Cancer. Learn what gave him the strength to carry on in Fight The Good Fight.

DEDICATION

This book is dedicated to former U.S.B.A. Middleweight Champion Alex Ramos and to all of the great warriors of boxing that are suffering from the effects of pugilistic dementia (the medical term for being "punch drunk").

These fighters gave their heart and soul to the sport. Each walked that lonely walk, too many times, down the aisle of the arena, climbed those noble steps into the inner sanctum of the boxing ring, where only the strong survive. They were young, courageous, and powerful men who fought wars in the gym and in the arena not realizing they were mortal.

Then after the show is over, the cheering crowd gone, the fighter needs help to reach the dressing room, he has nothing left - his, energy, strength, and vitality completely spent in the ring. All he has left is courage, his body is riddled with pain, his face and hands are now swollen. He needs stitches above an eye and an X-ray of his hand. In the dressing room he sits and wonders why he gives so much and receives so little in return from the sport he has given his life to.

In a few weeks a boxing promoter will call and offer a fight. Boxing is in his blood, he can't quit. Another match will be made and the warrior will do it yet again.

The above scenario is exactly what goes on in many dressing rooms when the fight is over - so many of these men can't walk away from the sport. The roar of the crowd, the money, fame, a shot at the title become the addiction the fighter can't beat.

The career is over, the entourage is gone, and the fighter is by himself now. Depressed and alone the boxer seeks affirmation and a new identity. He's always been a fighter. That's all he knows. What can he do? What will he do? Such is the life of a professional boxer.

Many of these former professional athletes are now homeless and are battling a much tougher foe than the fiercest boxer they ever faced in the boxing ring.

These men need our prayers and our help. The Retired Boxer's Foundation is an organization whose sole purpose is to help retired boxers.

The retired Boxer's Foundation was founded by former U.S.B.A. champion Alex "The Bronx Bomber" Ramos in 1998. Ramos also suffers from the ravages of pugilistic dementia.

We salute Alex Ramos and all of the other brave combatants who have given so much to our beloved sport of boxing.

You may contact the Retired Boxer's Foundation at:

www.retiredboxers.org

Phone: (805) 955-9064

Table of Contents

ACKNOWLEDGMENTS

I want to thank Ryan Waldrop, Ronquillo Pacheo, Keith McKnight, Timmy Miller, Jake Thomas, Jonathon Reid, the rest of the Club Knockout team, and Christy Halbert of the Boxing Resource Center for helping in the development of the Pro Boxing Trainer, Training Program.

I'd like to thank Adam Richards, "Diamond" Jim MacDonald, "Dangerous" Don Wilford, Donald Bowers, Darryl "Fast Fists" Fuller, Ken "The Bull" Atkin, Keith McKnight, John "Buddy" West, Timmy Miller, Tim "Scrap Iron" Johnson, Chilsom Bobo, Warren "The Warrior" Williams, and also to the many amateur boxers who were a part of our team for allowing me to be a part of your careers. We traveled all over the world together and had a blast. Thanks for the memories.

I need to acknowledge the great trainers who helped us over the years Former Middleweight Contender Mark Frazier, Hall of Fame boxer Curtis Cokes, Jeff Thomas, Wrestling great Billy Robinson, Leroy Ozier, Rayford Collins, Ace Miller, the great Kronk trainer Luther Burgess, former heavyweight champion Big John Tate, and of course Benito Ortiz.

And I must thank Stephanie Boles, and my wife Lanita for taking the photos that illustrate the techniques in the book. You ladies, Rock!

ROUND 1

THE BOXER'S STANCE

"Once that bell rings you're on your own. It's just you and the other guy." -Joe Louis

Before you begin a boxing training program there are a few things you should know. The most basic of which is the boxer's stance or on guard position. If you stand squarely in front of your opponent at a 90 degree angle you will be an easy target for your foe to hit. You want to face your opponent at a 45 degree angle as you see demonstrated in the photo below. This makes you a harder target to hit. In reality you are positioning yourself sideways toward your opponent.

You want to keep your feet a shoulder width apart. If you are right handed you will face your opponent with your left foot forward as I demonstrate in the photo. This is called the orthodox or right handed stance. Your forward hand will be your lead or the hand that you jab with. In the next section you will learn that everything is set up by your jab - Everything.

If you are left handed you would stand the opposite way with your right shoulder facing your target. This is called the southpaw or left handed stance.

Elbows should be tucked securely next to your rib-cage and both of your hands should be held high enough to protect your face. With your elbows and forearms tucked securely around your body you won't need to worry about your opponent's body shots. A good body puncher can break your ribs or drop you with a crushing hook to the liver. The number one rule in boxing is to protect yourself at all times.

I teach new boxers to hold their hands next to their cheekbones for protection. As you gain experience and learn to block and slip punches you can carry your hands a little lower.

Note in the photo that my rear heel is lined up with my front toe. Both feet are pointed at a 45 degree angle. My knees and hips are slightly bent and my back is pretty straight.

You will also notice that my rear heel is off of the floor. This acts as a shock absorber if I get hit and it keeps me on balance. When a boxer is in this stance he will not stagger if pushed. He is coiled and ready to strike his target just like a King Cobra.

Once you climb into the boxing ring you are on your own. The referee is there to see that your opponent doesn't break the rules.

Your trainer is in the corner to give you instructions, but you are on your own. This is a "hurt" sport. Your opponent is in the hurting business and you need to understand that before you climb into the boxing ring.

I'm writing this to help you learn how to protect yourself. I'm sharing the things I've learned as a professional boxing trainer of over twenty years. I never want to see anybody get hurt in the sport. I believe that a boxing match should be stopped too early instead of too late.

My advice to you is to make sure you are in great shape and ready to fight before you climb those four steps into the squared circle.

You can use euphemisms and say it's a sport. You can call it boxing instead of brawling or fighting. You can say it's an art form. You can say boxing is poetry in motion. And for people in the audience, those outside the ring, it is a sport. This is a boxing match for them because they aren't getting hit. They paid money to watch two gladiators try to kill each other.

Boxer's Stance

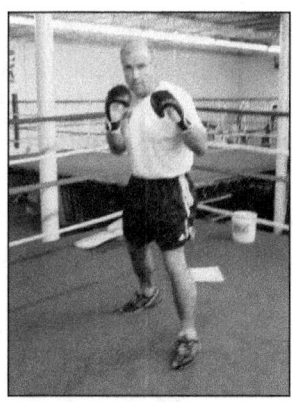

But they aren't pouring their heart and soul out in the ring. You are. They aren't putting up their own hide, blood, sweat and tears like you. For the boxer this is a fight, this is hand to hand combat, this is war. And many times a boxer has to fight for his life. This is a blood sport and don't ever get into the ring and take it lightly. The man or woman in the other corner is trying to hurt you; they are trying to knock you out. They are not your friend. They're your enemy.

When the contest is over you can help him/her up, hug their neck, and be their buddy. But never try to be their friend before you have fought them.

This sport is psychological warfare and if you try to be friendly with your opponent before the bout, they will think you are weak and are afraid of them.

Be stoic and never let anyone know what you are thinking. Don't show fear and you never want to show anger. An angry boxer is an easy boxer to beat. That probably sounds strange to you, but it's true.

An angry boxer is a tense fighter. He flexes his muscles before every punch so his opponent can easily see what he is about to do. His punches are stiff and his motion is awkward. Because of this I always tell my fighters ***"If you lose your temper, you lose the fight."***

Do not show emotion. You never want to show pain, certainly not fear, and you don't even want to smile. If we are boxing and you hit me in the ribs and you see that I am hurt. What is the first thing you are going to do? Exactly, you are going to hit me where it hurts.

Do not ever show when and where you are hurt. If you get hurt hold on to your opponent until you clear your head, the pain goes away, or the referee breaks you and your opponent. If you are still hurt hold your opponent again. The key is to hold without letting anyone know you are hurt until you are able to recover and get back into the fight.

You can't hold your opponent forever, otherwise you'll lose on a disqualification. But it's okay to clinch when you are hurt.

Some people will try to tell you to never hold your opponent, but I'm telling you like it is. Sometimes you get tagged and if you don't hold and hang on until you clear your head you could be knocked out.

On the other hand if you get into the ring and hold your opponent all of the time without fighting, you have no business being in the ring. This is called boxing, not holding.

So learn to fight well and give the fans a great show. But always remember to protect yourself and don't take any unnecessary punishment.

"Rhythm is everything in boxing. Every move you make starts with your heart, and that's in rhythm or you're in trouble." -Sugar Ray Robinson

"He went to the hospital with bleeding kidneys and me, I went dancing with my wife." -George Chuvalo after his 15 round loss to Muhammad Ali

"His mouth made him feel like he was gonna win. Not his hands, I had my hand. He had his lips." -Joe Frazier after his win over Muhammad Ali

"The attempt for greatness is the biggest drug in the world." -Mike Tyson

"Down goes Frazier! Down goes Frazier! Down goes Frazier!" -Howard Cosell after George Foreman put Frazier on the deck

"I hated every minute of training, but I said, "Don't quit. Suffer now and live the rest of your life as a champion." -Muhammad Ali

"It's not rage that drives me, it's competition." -Lennox Lewis

"I run miles out there on the road, long before I dance under those lights" -Muhammad Ali

Round 2

THE JAB

"It's hard to be humble when you're as great as I am" -
Muhammad Ali

Throughout the next few pages I'm going to explain boxing technique from the orthodox stance or from a right handed fighter's perspective. If you are a southpaw simply reverse the instructions that I teach and for the most part they work the same.

Boxing coach and former professional boxer Timmy Miller is demonstrating the left jab by punching a punch mitt or hand pad that I am holding in the photo below.

Left Jab

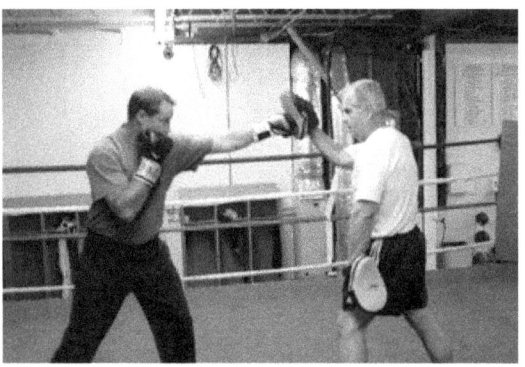

To execute the jab, start from the on guard position that you see in photo above and quickly step toward your target while shooting your left hand forward like a bullet being released from a gun. As your left hand snaps against your target quickly pronate your fist so that the palm of your hand faces downward. If thrown quickly and correctly you should hear a loud "pop" as your fist hits its intended target.

My good friend and professional boxing trainer Benito Ortiz was a Featherweight contender in the 1970's. After his professional boxing career, he was a noted house trainer at the famed Time Square Gym in the heart of downtown New York City. The gym was located a few blocks from Madison Square Garden and virtually everyone who fought at the Garden trained in the gym.

I often heard Benito ask fighters what was the very first thing they did when they arrived home to enter their house. Without fail each boxer would say **"Put the key in the door."** Benito would then tell the fighter that's what your jab is. It's the key to set up every punch you are going to throw. Your jab will set up your right cross, your left hook, and even your uppercut. Every combination begins with the jab.

Left Jab

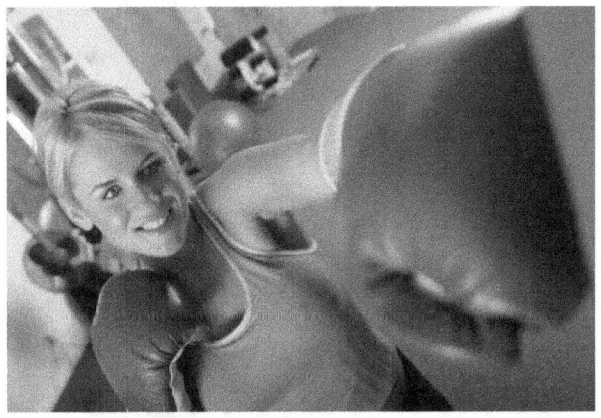

The jab is a great offensive weapon and it's a tremendous defensive tool. If you ever want to achieve anything in the sweet science of boxing, you must develop a world class jab.

I used to tell my boxers – *"jab when you are lonely, jab when you are blue, and jab when you don't know what to do."* Your jab is a fast long range missile that will determine how far you go or don't go in boxing. Your jab is also a short shotgun blast that can be thrown six inches and create an opening for the cross or hook.

Some people say that the jab is a weaker punch. I totally disagree. I've seen a properly thrown jab break a boxer's jaw, I've seen boxers get knocked out by a jab. A noted professional boxer broke my nose in a sparring session with a jab. And it was the most painful punch I ever felt in the ring. I still remember how it felt when it landed and that was in 1973. How would you like to develop a jab that is so good your adversary remembers it 40 years later?

You can throw a fast jab that has little power on it, but if you throw it properly your jab should snap like a whip as it strikes your target. And believe me if you get hit with a shot like that it hurts.

Muhammad Ali is said to have had the greatest jab in heavyweight history. But I absolutely loved how Larry Holmes, one of the most under rated champions of all time, threw his jab.

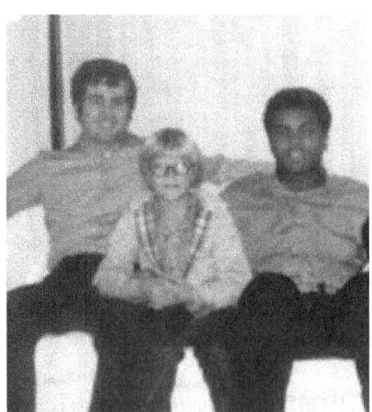

L-R Kerry, Todd Strachan, Muhammad Ali, 1971

Holmes could crush his opponent with his incredibly powerful jab, but he also used it as a steering wheel. He would maneuver his opponent to the left or right with his jab and maneuver his opponent into his cross or uppercut.

The great champion Tommy "Hit Man" Hearns would use his jab as a measuring rod. He would touch his opponent with that long jab and measure the distance that his deadly right hand needed to travel to crush his opponent's chin. Prelim fighters and legends alike felt the wrath of that Hearns jab. I saw it up close and personal as my boxer, Ken "The Bull" Atkin fought the great champion and I worked in the corner opposite Hearns team.

We trained Atkin for eight weeks to roll his shoulder and get away from that devastating right hand that the Hit Man was noted for. Every time Tommy threw the jab Atkin would slip to the right and roll the shoulder away from the right hand.

Although the legendary champion hit Atkin with crushing left hooks to the body and lightning fast jabs to the head, he didn't land his famous widow maker. Atkin was very competitive in the fight until he was severely cut above the eye and the fight was stopped in the third round. I uploaded a video of the entire bout to YouTube. Feel free to go to my channel (Kerry Pharr Boxing) on YouTube to watch it.

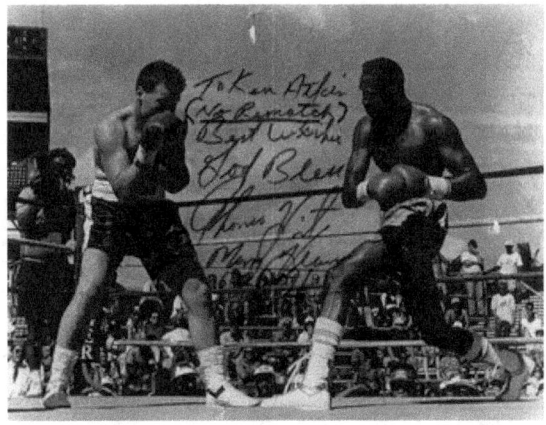

Atkin – Hearns

The power jab or shotgun jab actually gets its devastating force from your rear foot. Remember you back heel is raised two or three inches in the air. Notice legend Hearns rear heel in the photo. That's exactly the way it should be.

As you prepare yourself to fire your jab, you initiate the punch by explosively pushing you body forward from your rear foot. As your body moves forward you simultaneously shoot your left hand like water from a pressure washer toward your target.

As you extend your left arm you twist your fist (pronate) or turn it over. The arm should snap like a rubber band and crack like a whip on contact. There should be a small explosion as your punch lands. If it's executed correctly you'll hear a small explosion as it lands.

As important as a left jab is, you want to make sure you bring your left hand immediately back to guard your face. Many times a boxer will jab and draw his hand back to his waist. A smart opponent will counter punch with his right hand and if you do not bring your left hand back to the on-guard position you could be knocked out.

I always taught my boxers to counter their rival's jab by following the jab home with their right hand. After your opponent throws his jab at you and starts to pull his left hand back - you quickly throw your right hand towards his face. If he brings the jab hand back to his waist you will clip him on the chin with your counter punch.

After you throw any punch you must always - "without fail" bring your hands back to the on-guard position to protect yourself. As an old trainer friend of mine used to say *"Keep your guards up."*

If you would like to see this demonstrated on video please go to www.ProBoxingTrainer.com and register and I'll send you some **FREE** online boxing lessons.

"If you screw things up in tennis, it's 15 love, if you screw up in boxing it's your ass." -Randall "Tex" Cobb

"The three toughest fighters I ever fought were Sugar Ray Robinson, Sugar Ray Robinson and Sugar Ray Robinson. I fought Sugar so many times, I'm surprised I'm not diabetic. -Jake LaMotta

"To see a man beaten not by a better opponent but by himself is a tragedy." -Cus D'Amato

"From nothing to everything is a long way… From everything to nothing is one stop." -Wladimir Klitschko

ROUND 3

THE RIGHT CROSS

"I came from a dirt farm, now I'm filthy rich." -Larry Holmes

The right hand should never be thrown as a lead punch. You should always lead with your jab. Your left foot and left hand are the closest things to your target. You right hand or power hand is the farthest hand from your target. It has to travel a greater distance to hit your opponent. If you lead with your right hand and miss your opponent you will be wide open for a counter left hook.

The great fighters with blazing hand speed Ali, Leonard, Hearns and Jones could get away with throwing pot shots at their opponents with right hands leads. Most boxers cannot and it is very, very, dangerous to lead with a right hand unless you are counter punching. But that's a different story because your opponent has taken the initiative to lead and has committed his jab so you can counter with your right hand because he's not in position to hit you with his hook.

Right Cross

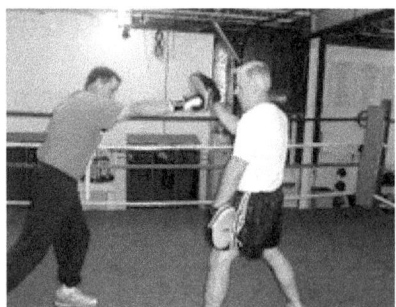

The first action is to push off of your back foot which generates the power to land your jab. After you hit your target with your jab and begin the process of pulling the jab back to cover your chin, you rotate your right shoulder, lean to your left almost like you are doing a side bend and throw your straight right hand across the jab. You will never hit your left arm but you want to throw your straight right cross over your extended jab. As you twist your body, your left hand will naturally return to your left side as you throw your cross.

The straight right hand or right cross is thrown immediately after the left jab. As you bring your left hand back to guard your face you release the right hand. As the punch lands, you will twist your right foot to increase the power of the blow. This is the classic one-two punch combination. Notice how the right side of Timmy's chin is covered (in the photo) with his shoulder to guard against a counter left hook.

The Slam or Slammer

Often you will hear someone talk about a right hook in boxing. And from the orthodox stance (right handed) there is really no right hook. A right hook is thrown by a southpaw boxer from the left-handed stance.

The reason for the confusion is that there is a punch in boxing called the slam or slammer that is thrown very similar to a hook. We'll explain the hook in detail in the next chapter.

After you land a right cross or a straight right hand, if you are close to your opponent, you can slam a right hand behind his guard.

Once you are close to you opponent, usually you are so close to your opponent that you are both fighting inside, place your left shoulder on your opponent's chest and throw your right hand behind your opponent's left glove. You want to make sure your wrist is bent and that your fist is perpendicular or vertical and throw it behind his glove. Again you have to be very careful because in essence you are throwing a right hand lead. The only difference is that you are close to your opponent's chest and aren't throwing the right hand from long range. But a good fighter can still counter punch you so be sure to bring your hand back or squat to avoid the counter hook.

The Overhand Right

The overhand right is a deadly punch and often leads to a knockout when it lands cleanly. Most fighters use their left jab to set up power punches and since this punch is a right hand and travels such a long distance it can open you up to a left hook counter if you lead with this punch. This punch is normally delivered behind the adversary's left glove and often lands on the temple, ear, mouth or nose.

To execute this punch the weight should be on the ball of your right foot. Spin your right heel and rotate your right shoulder and hips toward your target while dipping to your left side. This punch is an arcing punch, not a straight shot like the right cross.

If you perfect this technique you can use it as a deadly counter over your opponent's left jab. Two of the most devastating knockouts I ever saw were by one of the professional boxers on our team. This boxer was an extremely tough boxer. He was so tough that we called him Scrap Iron. He was a brawler and not a puncher. Throughout his entire boxing career he only knocked out a few of his opponents.

One of these happened in the gym while he was a teenager and the other in a professional boxing match. Both of these scary knockouts happened because Scrap Iron had a wild, vicious, overhand right and if it landed somebody was bound to get hurt.

Our young team was training in a baseball announcer's building that the mayor of the city we lived in, allowed us to use as a gym. It was a small cinder block building with a carpeted wooden floor upstairs that we roped off and used as a boxing ring. We had about 20 young men who were learning how to box in the building.

A tall, rugged fellow by the name of Lonnie was training with us. Lonnie was about 21 years old. He didn't follow instructions well. In fact, he wouldn't do anything I asked him to do. Each time I let him spar he tried to murder his sparring partner.

I never allowed one boxer to abuse another. Since the guys were boxing and hitting each other, obviously someone would get clipped on the chin and would get knocked down or knocked out. But that was a rare occasion. The boxers always wore protective gear, and we were careful not to let things get out of control in practice. They would spar in 16-ounce training gloves, wear a headgear, a protective cup and a mouthpiece.

I was a relatively young coach and didn't handle the following situation very well. I was trying to teach Lonnie and the other fellows how to box. I normally worked with a double end bag and speed bag before I would allow them to begin "controlled sparring." We would put sparring gloves on two boxers of the same age, weight and skill level and I would allow them to spar with each other using only the jab.

The jab is the most important punch a boxer learns. It isn't the most powerful punch, but it is usually the most effective punch. A boxer always leads with a jab. It sets all the other punches up. Former world heavyweight champion Larry Holmes dominated the division for seven years, largely on the strength of his great left jab. Holmes realized that to control an opponent in a match, you have to establish the jab first. For a right-handed boxer, the left jab is the lead but the right hand, the left hook and the uppercut are the power punches. The jab is the first punch that you teach to a new boxer.

Lonnie was sparring with another boxer and the other youngster, as instructed, was using only his jab. Even though I had asked Lonnie to use only his left jab, Lonnie threw wild right hands and screamed at his sparring partners, intentionally trying to hurt them. I was frustrated and angry with him and I could see that I was going to have to put someone else with experience in to spar with Lonnie.

So I gloved Scrap Iron up, who was then 19, and whispered in his ear, *"I want you to teach this kid a lesson."*

Both of the boxers were gloved and ready to spar. When the bell rang to begin the round, Lonnie let out a blood-curdling scream and charged across the ring toward Scrap Iron. I believe that it actually scared Scrap Iron, and out of fear he threw an incredibly vicious wild right hand that landed squarely on Lonnie's mouth.

Lonnie crashed to the floor, and the building shook like we were in an earthquake. Scrap Iron knocked Lonnie out cold; he was bleeding from the mouth where the punch had caused a tooth to puncture his lip. His face was as white as a ghost and he looked seriously hurt. It was a very scary moment for me and I turned to Scrap Iron and said, *"Gees Scrap, I didn't mean for you to kill him!"*

Jimmy Brindley, another boxer, was standing by watching the sparring. Seeing Lonnie get knocked out so viciously scared Jimmy so much that he immediately took off his gloves, left the boxing gym and never returned.

He later told another boxer, *"Man, he hit him so hard I saw the light. That's the end of my boxing career."*

About 15 or 20 seconds later Lonnie came to. He needed a few stitches in his mouth, but other than his pride being hurt he was OK. I don't know why, but he never returned to the gym either.

Former heavyweight champion James "Bone crusher" Smith had a devastating overhand right. Smith told me that his trainer and former world welterweight champion Emile Griffin instructed him to land his right hand on his opponent's ear and drive him to the canvas. And he did so with a vengeance when he demolished former ex-world champ Mike Weaver in one round and won the biggest prize in all of sports - the heavyweight championship of the world - by crushing WBA champ Tim Witherspoon. That overhand right was so powerful it smashed Witherspoon to the canvas three times in the first round.

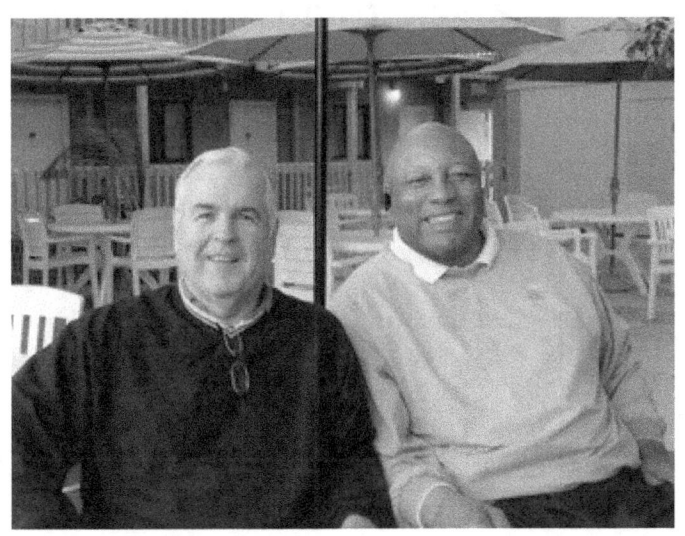

Kerry - James "Bone crusher" Smith

Round 4

The Left Hook

"Boxing is the only sport you can get your brain shook, your money took and your name in the undertaker book." -Joe Frazier

It was dubbed the Fight of the Century and it was the first boxing match between Joe Frazier and Muhammad Ali. Joe Frazier was 26-0 with 23 KOs and the former champion, now challenger Muhammad Ali, had recently returned from a three year forced layoff from boxing for refusing to be inducted into the United States Army. Ali was 31-0 with 25 KOs.

The fight lived up to its hype and went the entire 15-round championship distance. Early in round 15, Frazier landed what might have been the most spectacular left hook ever thrown in boxing. The punch not only put the great Muhammad Ali on his back it almost flipped him over backwards as he crashed to the ring canvas. This was the only fight that Frazier would win in their trilogy and he did it with heart, skill, and an unbelievably powerful left hook.

The left hook is one of the most devastating punches in the sport of boxing. When it is thrown correctly and lands squarely on an opponent's chin a knockout usually occurs.

There are a variety of ways to throw the punch. Many trainers teach the boxer to shift his body weight to the rear, or supporting foot, permitting him to pivot his front foot and torso toward his opponent as he throws his fist horizontally toward his target. In this scenario the left elbow is brought up almost parallel to the floor so that the arm forms an L shape as the punch is delivered. The palm of the hand is facing the floor.

My preference is to throw the hook similar to the way the great Joe Frazier did which is the opposite way of what I just described to you. A good way to practice this hook is to stand in your traditional on guard boxing stance. Push off of your rear foot and step forward with your left foot. As your weight bottoms out on your left side spin your heel to the left and shift your body to the right very quickly powerfully delivering your left hook to your target.

If you will look at the photo below you will note that I have shifted my weight to my left side to catch Timmy's hook, but I'm also in the perfect position to throw my hook. My weight is on my left leg and if I wanted to I could raise my left elbow upward and throw my hook.

To execute the punch shift your weight to your left side, the left elbow is brought up almost parallel to the floor so that the arm forms a hook shape (note left hook photo); your left palm should be facing your face, pivot on the ball of your left foot and spin your left heal outward while your left leg and torso turn sharply to the right. Punch through your target instead of to your target. You always want to punch through your target. If you have ever played billiards you know how to put "English" on the ball. When throwing your hook try to put a little "English" or snap on the end of the delivery.

Left Hook

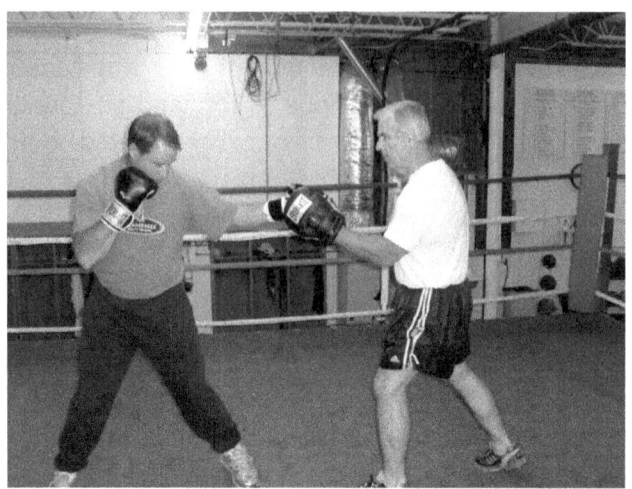

I always taught my boxers to rotate the hand so that your palm is perpendicular to your face and bend the wrist toward your body. If you looked at your hand while throwing this hook the palm of your hand, your four fingers and your thumb would be facing you.

Almost everybody else teaches that your palm should face the floor when you execute the hook. You can throw it anyway you wish but I believe that you will be able to generate much more power with the hook I've just described than the other variations.

Try different ways to throw all of your punches and see which works best for you.

"I used to be a middleweight, now all my weight is in the middle." - Mark Frazier

"Earnie Shavers could punch you in the neck and break your ankle" -Randall "Tex" Cobb

ROUND 5

THE UPPERCUT

"He can have the heart, he can hit harder and he can be stronger, but there's no smarter fighter than me." -Floyd Mayweather

My former boxing trainer used to call this punch an upper shoot. It is and has always been referred to in boxing as an upper-cut.

The right uppercut is a very powerful punch that is thrown inside when you are very close to your opponent. If you attempt to throw this punch from the outside you will not land the punch and almost certainly will get hit by a counter left hook.

The uppercut is thrown upward and directed underneath the chin or into the solar plexus.

Uppercut

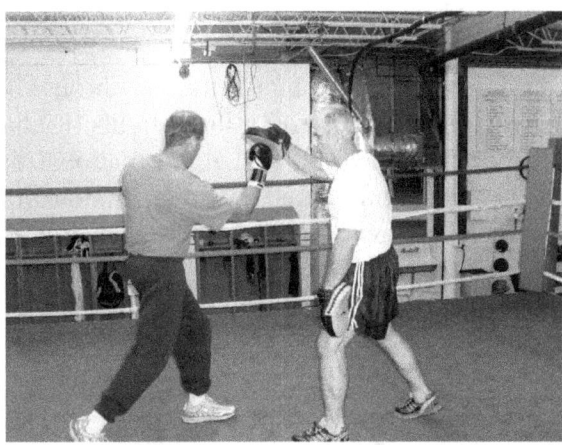

To throw a right uppercut, start in your boxing stance with the back (right) knee bent. Lower the right shoulder to drop the right side of the body in a semi-crouch position. Keep your left fist up by your chin to protect the head. Now as you rotate the hips forward, push the ball of the back foot, (the right foot), and punch the right fist up towards the target. Remember that this is a punch that should only be thrown while you are fighting inside.

I've often seen boxers try to throw this punch straight up toward their adversary's chin and miss the chin entirely. The better way to throw this punch is to open the arm up so that there is a six to eight inch gap between your chin and your fist. Aim the punch at your opponent's chest and once it hits his chest it will slide upward and clip him underneath his chin.

If you hold your hand too close to your chin and aim for your adversary's chin the only thing you'll end up hitting is thin air or yourself. You will miss your target completely.

A true uppercut is thrown from the right hand. You will sometimes hear people refer to a left uppercut. You can throw the left hand in a similar fashion to an uppercut and for the lack of a better term we will call it an uppercut.

Adam Richards was a boxer that I trained throughout his amateur career and for his first three professional fights. Richards had a very powerful left hook and he won four junior national titles and fought for the cruiserweight professional world championship mostly on the strength of that great hook. He and Mike Tyson co-hold the junior Olympic record of each winning two national junior Olympic titles and knocking out each and every opponent that they faced en route to each national championship.

Richards was very effective with his left hand. He was a shorter heavyweight similar to Tyson. Richards would land the left hook and immediately shoot the punch upward in the same manner you would throw an uppercut. When Richard landed the punch the fight was over.

Keith McKnight was a world class heavyweight that I trained throughout his amateur and professional careers. McKnight is six foot, six inches tall and a very fast, mobile and crafty boxer.

McKnight was so tall and fast that he could hit an opponent with a left jab and immediately turn his left hand into a vicious uppercut which would lift the opponent's head into the air allowing McKnight to throw his right cross over the top and knock his adversary out all in about one second of time.

McKnight's sugar stick combination was a very fast jab, a left uppercut with the same hand, and a right cross to close the show. Imagine getting hit with three punches like that all in one second from a heavyweight fighter. Seeing a gifted boxer throw a combination such as this is a thing of beauty to watch but not to be on the receiving end of.

It worked well enough for McKnight to finish his career with a record of 44 wins and 4 losses- including a win over former world title challenger Phil Jackson and knockout wins over former world champions J.B. Williamson and Iran Barkley.

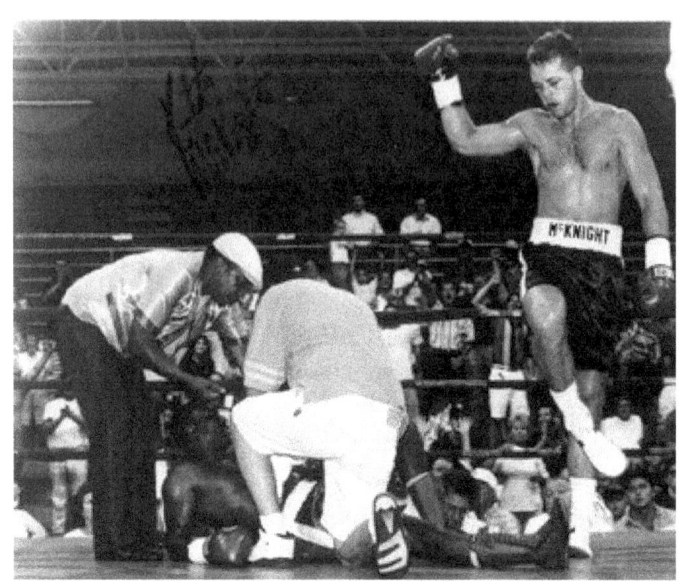

McKnight

ROUND 6

FANCY FOOTWORK

"Float like a butterfly, sting like a bee." -Muhammad Ali

Before you can float like a butterfly and sting like a bee you have to get comfortable in your stance and learn to glide around the ring like you are on ice skates.

Muhammad Ali had great mobility and in the early part of his career he was nearly impossible to hit as he danced around the ring like gravity didn't apply to him.

A boxer with great mobility is like poetry in motion. He is very graceful and entertaining to see.

Ali was once asked if he could have beaten Mike Tyson when both of them were in their prime. Without hesitation he replied- *"Yes, because you see I was a dancer."* Of course he was referring to his great mobility and the fact that Tyson wasn't known for movement. He had tremendous speed and crushing power, but not mobility.

A fighter who can't move is like a man stuck in quicksand (I'm not referring to Tyson, he wasn't mobile, but he was very fast, and he could jump on an opponent and knock him out in a flash).

If you have great mobility it is easy to beat a fighter who can't move, or one whose feet are stuck in quicksand. All you have to do is hit your opponent as you move in and out and side to side, without allowing him to hit you. Game over. No contest.

Once you are comfortable in your stance you can begin to move forward, backward, left or right.

As you move forward push off of your right foot, but step first with your left foot. When moving backward push backward with your front foot but move your rear foot first. When moving to the left your left foot is your lead foot. When moving right, move your right foot first. Drag the second foot back into position. I always instructed the boxers to "push, drag." You push one foot as you step and then you drag the other foot into position.

Pivoting

From your stance you can easily pivot around your opponent. Just raise the heel on your forward foot and pivot to the right or left 45 degrees and you will be behind your opponent in a position to strike him without him being able to strike you.

You can also pivot right and or left and glide around the ring on your toes.

Mobility Drill

If you have access to a boxing ring and you would like to learn how to glide around the ring like a ballerina here's a drill you can use to learn this skill.

Place you back against the ring ropes and get into your boxing stance. Start moving to your right. Push off of your left foot and allow your right foot to go first. Push, drag, push, drag while you are gliding toward the corner post. When you reach the corner - STOP! Then pivot to your right and glide down to the next corner - STOP! Pivot again.

After you worked on that move for a while move the other way by pushing off of the right foot and allowing the left foot to go first. Glide to the end of the ring and -STOP! Pivot left and keep going.

It is very difficult to teach someone proper boxing technique from a book. I have over 100 training videos to help you learn these skill sets. If you would like to receive some Free training videos that explain this in detail please go to www.ProBoxingTrainer.com and simply put in your name and email address and I'll send seven training videos to you.

Additionally if you are already a boxer and you are having trouble learning any of these things feel free to contact us. We occasionally have boxer's training camps and we would be delighted to work with you. You will get the benefit of working with professional boxing trainers who can help you improve your skill level.

Keith McKnight was a very mobile heavyweight and a slick boxer as well. He and I taped several videos together where he shows you how to glide effortlessly around the ring. If you want to learn ring generalship and mobility you need to see McKnight in action. I uploaded several of his bouts to YouTube. Once you are on YouTube just type in Kerry Pharr Boxing and all of those videos will come up.

"I was knocking guys out in the streets before I knew how to throw a jab and keep your chin down." -Bernard Hopkins

"I wish I would have knocked him out but I'll take the win." - Sugar Shane Mosley

"I have to accept the result from the fight and move on with my career." -Juan Manuel Marquez

"I started to work on him with the first ring of the bell. It wasn't an easy fight, It was a tough fight. -Miguel Cotto

"Trust me, he is not going to go 12 rounds with me." -Roy Jones Jr.

"What's your excuse tonight Roy." -Antonio Tarver

ROUND 7

HOW TO BLOCK PUNCHES

"Sure the fight was fixed. I fixed it with a right hand." -George Foreman

Your first line of defense is a good solid stance with your hands held close to you face and your elbows tucked tightly against your ribs. Some fighters learn a little bit about the sport and they think they are cute. They want to be a hot dog so they drop their hands and stick their chin or even their tongue out at their opponent. Over the years I've observed that this is a good way to get knocked out.

Just before the opening bell rang for every match I always told my boxers - *"Keep your hands up, your chin down, and your butt off of the canvas."* This statement is somewhat humorous, but it is true. If you keep your hands up and your chin down you are very unlikely to get hit with a clean punch that would knock you down or out. And it's very embarrassing to pick yourself up off of the boxing ring's canvas floor.

I mentioned my fighter Scrap Iron earlier. Scrap Iron for whatever reason thought he was a pretty boy and he often put his hands by his side and stuck his chin out and dared his opponent to hit him.

I was in Recife, Brazil with Scrap Iron and he was fighting Luciano Torres for the WBF super-middleweight world championship.

While the promoter was taking us around the city for press conferences and interviews we stopped at an open air market, a city block in size, with a tin roof and no walls. Scrap Iron began to run his mouth and the local butcher was offended. He came from behind his counter with a meat cleaver and started towards our group threatening us with his cleaver.

Although Scrap Iron didn't learn his lesson in this instance, he wisely closed his mouth and we escaped without harm.

The fight was the next day. The venue was a bull ring filled with 5,000 Brazilians all rabid, seemingly lunatic, fans of Luciano Torres. Scrap Iron was out boxing and out foxing the Brazilian that the locals called Todo Duro, which I'm told means hard as steel in their native Portuguese. As the fight progressed Scrap Iron began to put his hands down by his side and started sticking his chin out daring Todo Duro to hit him.

The locals went berserk and began to throw oranges and cups and everything else they could find into the ring. This only emboldened Scrap Iron who then began to stick his tongue out at Torres taunting him even more. His opponent and the fans were hysterical they wanted blood and I was wondering if we would be able to escape alive, let alone in one piece.

Scrap Iron wasn't protecting himself, he got careless and in the 7th round Torres caught him with a good shot over his left eye. Scrap Iron was cut and the fight was stopped in the 8th round. This was Scrap Iron's last shot at a world title and he let it slip away because of carelessness.

The lesson here is to keep your hands up, your chin down to protect yourself and don't get cute in the boxing ring.

The Parry

The first defensive hand technique that I teach boxers is the parry. I call it a pick. When your opponent jabs toward your face, open your right hand slightly until it forms a cup shape. As the jab nears your face push the right hand to your left in a short catching motion and parry the jab away from you. It sounds difficult but it is pretty easy to learn. You won't be able to pick every jab but it will help deflect most of them.

Future champ Ryan Waldrop is demonstrating How to Pick a Jab.

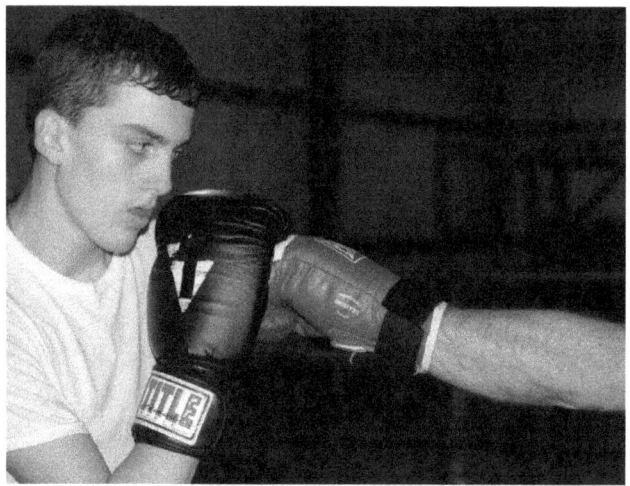

Ryan Waldrop picking a jab

One of the easiest ways to counter your opponent's jab is to pick it as you see Ryan demonstrating in the above photo and then immediately stick your jab in his face. I call this technique "Pick and Stick". Pick his jab then stick your jab.

Picking a Right Cross

If you are quick you can also pick/parry your competitor's right cross with your left hand. It is executed exactly like the right hand pick only in the opposite direction.

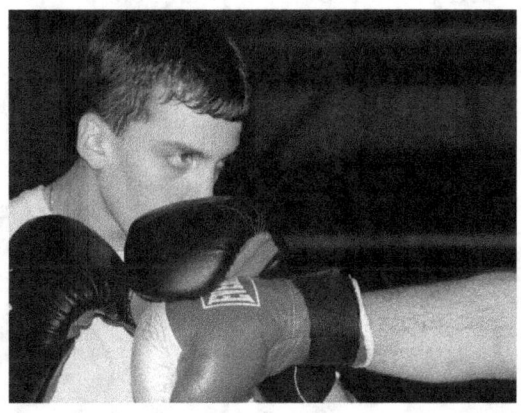

Right cross parry

Blocking a Right Cross

You can also block your opponent's right cross by raising your left hand and touching your forehead or ear. Push outward ever so slightly with your glove as you feel the punch connect. Do not let your glove touch your head. As a young boxer I let my glove hit my head while sparring, trying to block punches. After training I was getting headaches. I asked my trainer about it and he told me to stop the punch in mid-air before it hits your head. Resist the punch with your left hand, don't let it crash against your head.

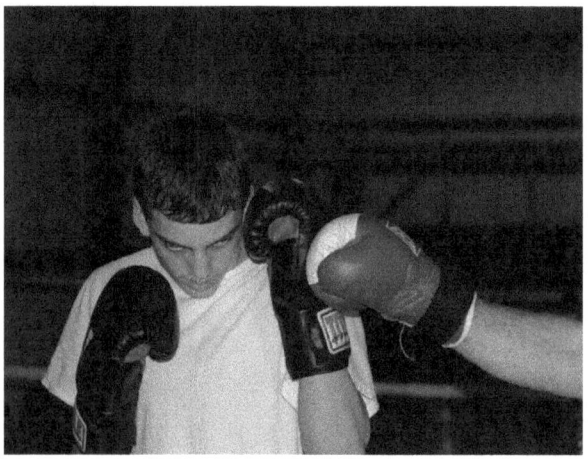

Blocking Right Cross

Catching an Uppercut

To stop a right uppercut from landing on your chin drop you open right hand on top of the punch and catch it just like you are catching a ball in a glove.

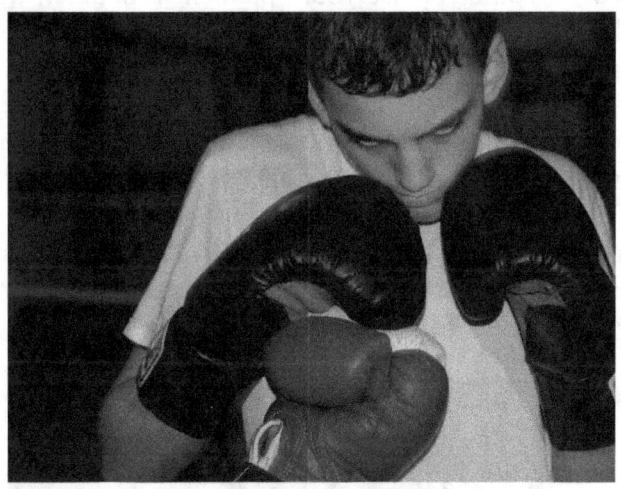

Catching uppercut

Blocking a Left Hook

Whenever you see your opponent square his shoulders, he is getting ready to launch a left hook at you. All fighters fight out of a 45 degree stance and in order to throw a hook a boxer has to square his shoulders. Anytime you see your opponent's shoulders at a 90 degree angle or whenever he is facing you squarely be prepared he's positioning himself to throw the left hook.

Once you see him throw the hook you can squat down and bob to your right to get underneath the punch. Or you can block the hook by raising your right hand to your ear and catching it on the outside of your hand before it lands on your face. I've been hit in the face and I've been hit in the hand by a left hook. Trust me, catching it on your hand feels a lot better than having it bash your face.

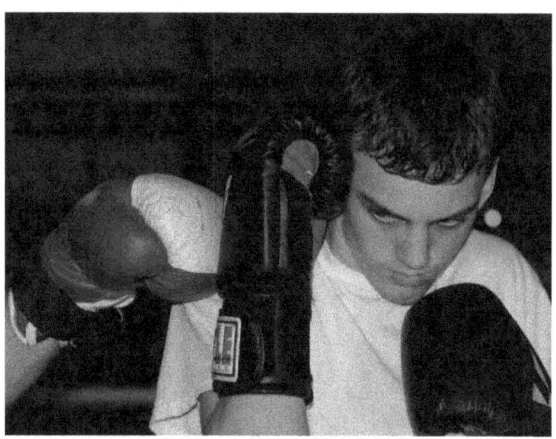

Ryan Blocking a Left Hook

"If I survived the Marines, I can survive Ali." -Chuck Wepner

"It's like someone jammed an electric light bulb in your face, and busted it. I thought half my face was blown off… When he knocked me down I could have stayed there for three weeks." -James J Braddock, after losing the heavyweight title to Joe Louis via knockout

"The question isn't at what age I want to retire, it's at what income." -George Foreman

"No mas." -Roberto Duran

ROUND 8

HOW TO SLIP PUNCHES

"Everybody's got plans... until they get hit." -Mike Tyson

From your boxing stance you will see the left jab coming straight toward your face. To slip a jab you bend sharply and quickly to your right side. Move just enough to avoid the punch. At that point you can roll underneath the jab and bob back to your left side and counter punch your opponent with your left hook.

To slip a right hand you bend to your left outside of the approaching right cross while turning your right shoulder toward your foe's chest. You will see Timmy Miller demonstrating how to slip punches in the figure below.

Tyson slip drill

The great boxing trainer Cus D'amato taught his champion boxers Floyd Patterson, Jose Torres and Mike Tyson a peek-a-boo style of defense that required a lot of practice at slipping punches.

Mike Tyson was the most famous of the champions and he worked regularly with a makeshift slipping bag hanging from a rope or chain to perfect his slipping technique. Subsequently this drill became known as the Tyson slip drill.

To do the Tyson slip bag drill you will need a small balloon or bag filled with sand (you can make your own). The bag is hanging from the ceiling with a small rope. Start by pushing the bag away from you like you would push a swing. As the bag nears your face move your head "slip" to the right or to the left to avoid being hit. Notice the blur behind Timmy's head. That is the slip bag as it passes over his right shoulder. This is one of the ways fighters practice to not get hit.

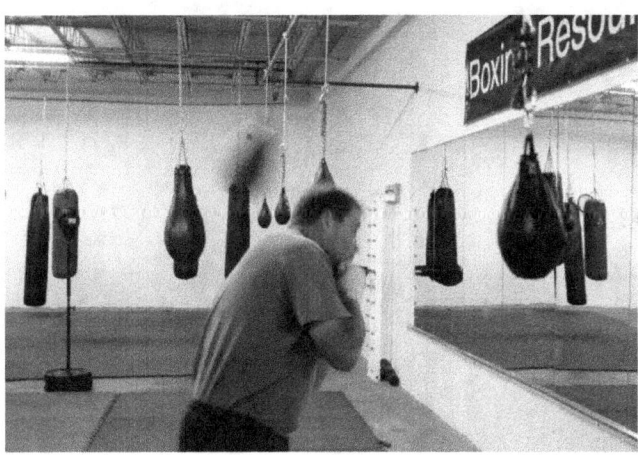

Slip Bag Drill

"I don't fight for legacy. I don't fight for none of that, I fight for that check. I'm in the check cashing business." -Floyd Mayweather Jr.

"Nothing personal - I am just doing my job." -Manny Pacquiao

"Why waltz with a guy for 10 rounds if you can knock him out in one?" -Rocky Marciano

"Hey, Ma, your bad boy did good!" -Rocky Graziano

"Boxing was not something I truly enjoyed. Like a lot of things in life, when you put the gloves on, it's better to give than to receive." -Sugar Ray Leonard

ROUND 9

BOBBING AND WEAVING

"All the time he's boxing, he's thinking. All the time he was thinking, I was hitting him." -Jack Dempsey

Bobbing and Weaving

If you are shorter than most of your foes you should learn the art of bobbing and weaving.

Jack Dempsey was heavyweight champion of the world from 1919 to 1926. Dempsey was about six feet tall and weighed only 190 pounds during his prime. I actually had the pleasure of meeting him in 1973 when he was in his late seventies.

When Dempsey won the world championship he faced champion Jess Willard who, for that time in history, was a Behemoth. Willard was six foot six inches tall and weighed in at the 240 pound range. The press called the fight a modern day David and Goliath because of the tremendous size difference between the combatants.

While Dempsey was training for the bout he developed a style that enabled him to roll underneath Willard's jab and get close enough to hit the champion. This technique became known as the Dempsey roll or the Dempsey crouch. Dempsey used it so well against Willard that he knocked the then champion down seven times in the first round alone.

Dempsey continued his fierce assault of Willard and beat him so thoroughly that it was reported that Willard had suffered a broken jaw, broken ribs, several broken teeth and a number of fractures to his facial bones. To keep him from further injury or even death

Willard's corner men would not allow him to come out for the 4th round.

I share Dempsey's story with you to illustrate the point that Mark Twain made over 100 years ago. *"It's not the size of the dog in the fight, it's the size of the fight in the dog."*

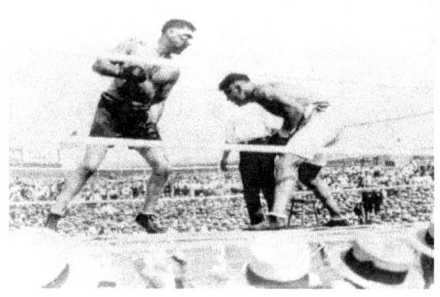

Willard - Dempsey 1919

Even though Dempsey was the smaller man he was much more of a fighter than the larger Willard. As a boxer you will meet fighters who are larger than you. Size doesn't always matter, but skill does and it helps to have techniques that allow smaller men to compete with bigger fighters. Bobbing and weaving is one of the best techniques to get underneath the punches of a taller fighter. The shorter fighter has a great advantage inside and underneath the taller fighter.

To execute this movement you will slip to the right outside of your opponent's jab and roll underneath back to the left. This is the Dempsey roll. You can also roll back and forth underneath your opponent's punches.

If you see a left hook coming toward your face squat down and roll underneath then outside and to your right rear. This will enable you to be in perfect position to counter with a right hand.

If your opponent throws a right hand at you, roll your left shoulder away from the punch, dip down and roll back inside underneath your adversary's assault. This will put you in position to counter with your left hook. If you wish to develop this skill I've explained how to do the bob and weave drill below.

Bob and Weave Drill

To utilize the bob and weave drill, you need a rope tied to two points at shoulder height. Begin in your boxing stance and bob left underneath the rope and then back to the other side. Each time you bob and weave step forward until you reach the end of your rope. Turn around and work your way back.

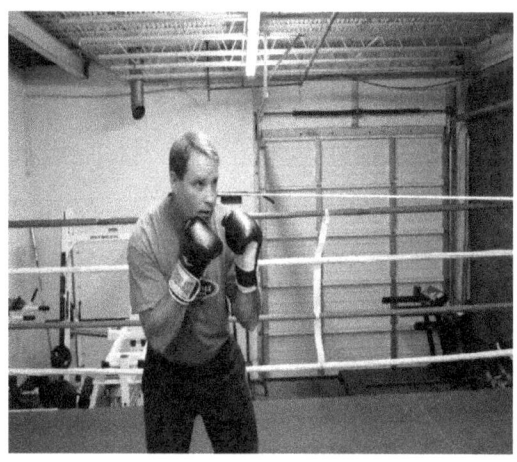

Bob and weave drill

ROUND 10

BOXER DRILLS = BOXER SKILLS

"Only in death will I relinquish my belts." -Manny Pacquiao

In the next few pages I'm going to share with you different tools you can use to develop you boxing technique. The first exercise is shadow boxing. Whenever you are shadow boxing you are punching at an imaginary opponent. This is an incredible way to improve your skill that doesn't require any equipment.

Shadow boxing

Stand in front of a mirror and begin to practice the punches and combinations you learned earlier. The person you see in the mirror is your imaginary opponent.

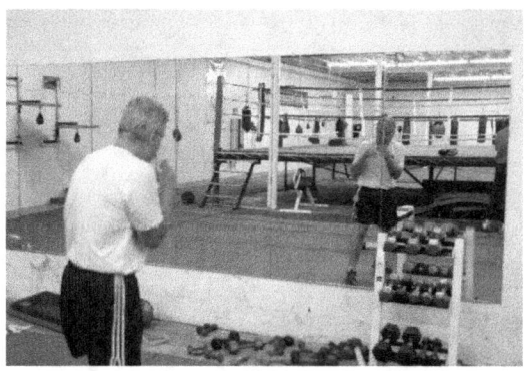

Shadow Boxing

Jumping Rope

The grand daddy of all gym exercises for boxers is jumping rope. Fighters usually jump rope for several rounds every day in the gym. I've seen fighters jump rope for an hour in a sweat suit attempting to make weight before a bout.

A jump rope will cost you less than $5 and it is one of the best exercises for improving conditioning and coordination.

To jump rope like a boxer you will first need to find a rope that is the ideal size for you. Today you can buy a plastic rope and adjust to fit your body. These inexpensive ropes are as good as or better than the old pro style leather ropes that were the standard in the boxing gym for years.

How to Skip

With your hands at your sides hold the rope handles lightly and turn them with your wrists in small circles. Keep your arms slightly bent and tilt your head down, but don't stare at your feet. Keep you upper body straight and erect and skip rope without jumping more than one inch off of the floor. Land on the balls of your feet, with your heels barely touching. Alternate back and forth from your left to right foot.

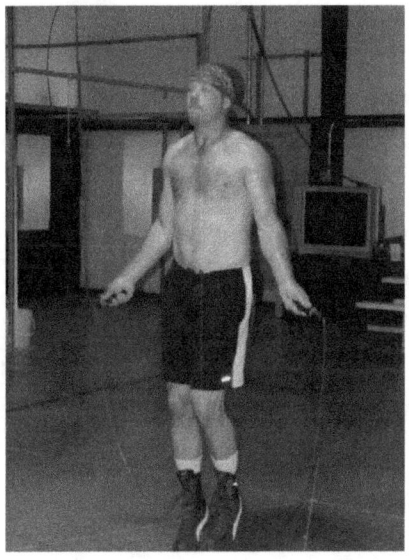

McKnight - Jump/Skip Rope

Heavy Bag Training

One of the most basic of all boxing exercises is punching the heavy bag. This exercise will shape and strengthen your whole body while improving cardio conditioning as well.

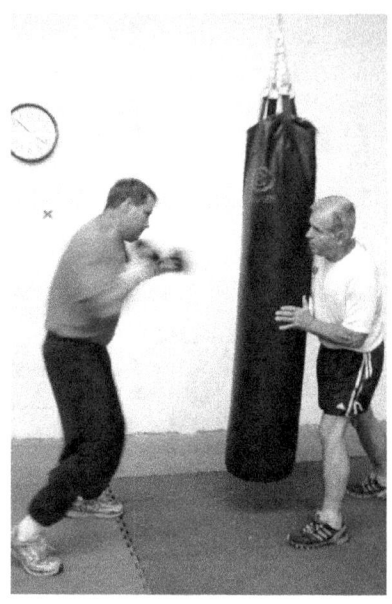

Heavy bag Work

After you warm up with two or three rounds of shadow boxing you want to move to the heavy bag. It's the long round bag that weighs about 100 pounds that you see in the gym.

Hit the bag and move to your left and right just like you are facing an opponent. As you hit the bag it will move allowing you the opportunity to work on your footwork at the same time you are improving your punching technique.

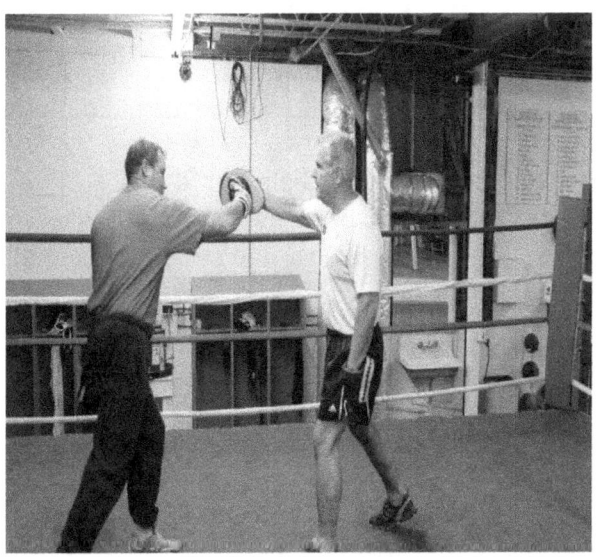

Punch mitt/hand pad work

Hand pad or punch mitt work

My favorite exercise in boxing is to hit or hold the hand pads for someone else. It is absolutely the best teaching tool for me in boxing. If you have a pair of punch mitts you can hold them for your training partner and they can do the same for you. I've worked 10 or 12 rounds with boxers on the pads who were getting ready for a big fight. In this illustration, Timmy is demonstrating the right hand slam.

Speed bag

Two of the boxing exercises that can make you look like a million dollars as a fighter are hitting the speed bag and jumping rope.

To hit the speed bag strike the bag with the face of your hand with a forward motion. As you strike the bag roll your hand in a circle toward you and then rotate it back to strike the bag, alternating right and left

Hands

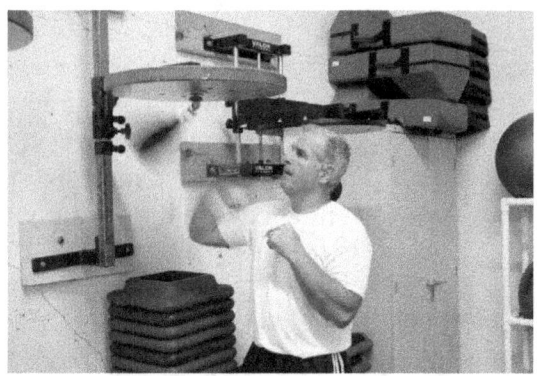

Speed bag

It takes a little time to learn how to hit the speed bag. Once you learn how, it helps you develop hand and eye coordination. It's hard to show some of these boxing exercises in a book so we have produced some FREE instructional videos to show you exactly how to do these exercises. Go to www.ProBoxingTrainer.com to see these videos.

Floor to ceiling bag

The floor to ceiling bag is a blur because Timmy just hit it. The bag has a rope attached to the top of it which is secured with a hook in the ceiling. There is a rubber strap from the bottom of the bag that is secured to the floor. Whenever you hit this bag it instantly recoils and snaps back at you. This is a great exercise for speed and timing. Notice the other floor to ceiling bags in the background.

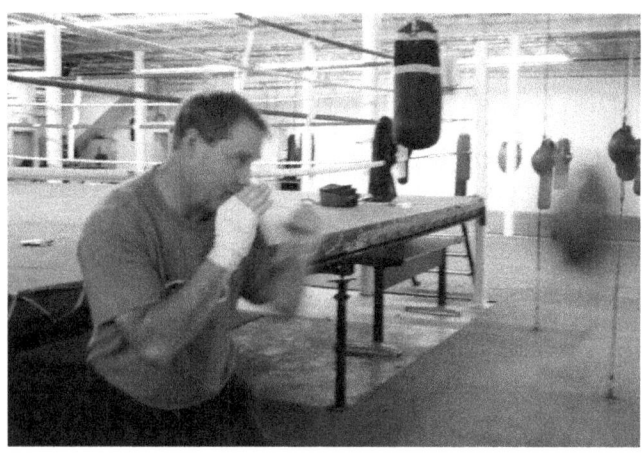

Floor to ceiling bag

"To be a successful boxer, the last thing you need to be doing is turning up to the gym stoned. You're going to get beaten up if you do that." -David Haye

"I love to knock guys out, that's my game." -Joe Calzaghe
"He can run, but he can't hide." -Joe Louis

"It's a mess. It's like it was 20 years ago before Mike Tyson cleaned things up. There really hasn't been a dominant heavyweight to come along since Lennox Lewis." -Emmanuel Steward

Touch him! Touch him! touch him! -Trainer Luther Burgess instructing a fighter on how to use his jab.

"Hit him. If he can take it, give it to him." -Luther Burgess

ROUND 11

HIGH INTENSITY TRAINING

"I don't care if you're a world champion six times over or a four round fighter who just got knocked out in 30 seconds of your first professional fight. To step inside that ring, you have to have guts."
-Oscar Dela Hoya

Marathon runners run long distances without any sudden bursts of speed. They have to pace themselves in order to complete their 26.2 mile race.

Boxers, on the other hand do not have the luxury of fighting at a slow pace. A boxer fights in explosive bursts and he or she needs to be in tremendous shape in order not to run out of gas during the fight. A tired fighter is an easy fighter to knock out.

One of the best conditioning exercises for a boxer is what we refer to as switches or burns. This is a high intensity conditioning workout that the boxer would normally do at the end of his regular workout after he is already tired.

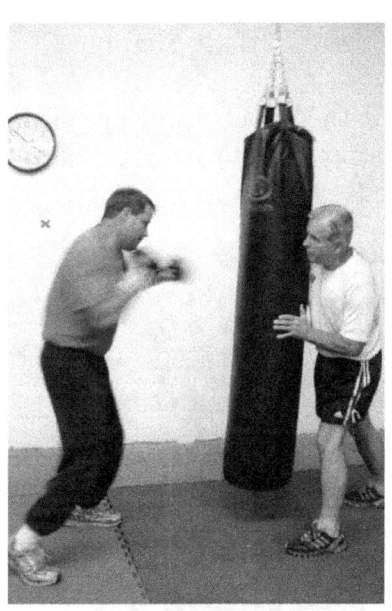

Heavy bag switches

In this exercise your workout partner holds the heavy bag or hand pads for you. You begin punching with 1-2 punch combinations as hard and as fast you can. You do this for 30 seconds and switch turns to allow your partner to punch the same way for 30 seconds while you hold the bag for them. Take alternate turns hitting the bag for 30 seconds for the full 3 minute round. Do three or four rounds of this everyday and you will be in championship shape in no time.

Body Shaping

After you have finished your warm up, medium and high intensity work, it's time to move on to body conditioning and body shaping work.

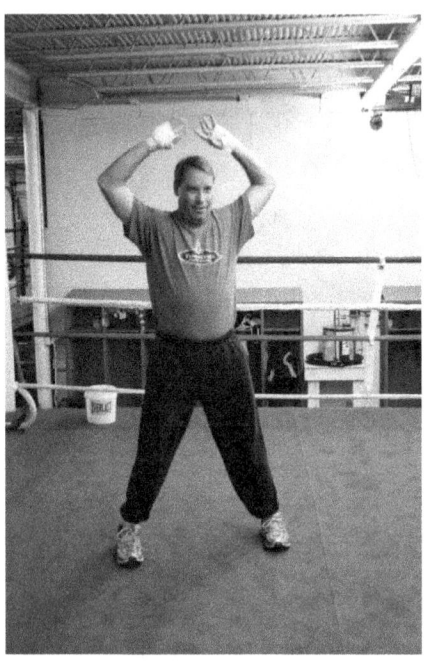

Jumping Jacks

Everybody loves jumping jacks. Jump in the air and spread your feet at the same time as you clap your hands together over your head.

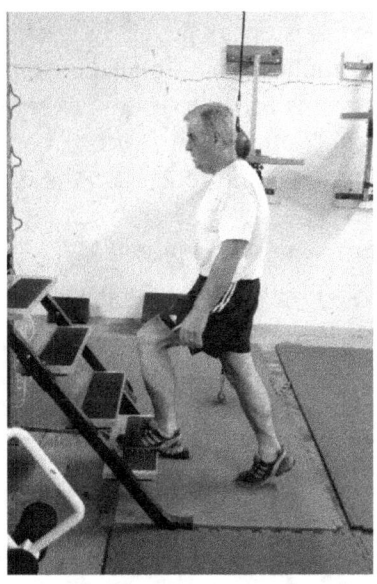

Step-ups

I learned this great exercise from hall of fame Wrestler Billy Robinson while he trained shoot or submission wrestlers in our gym.

Ideally you want your step to be 15-18 inches in height. A normal step is only about 9 inches. The higher the step the more difficult and beneficial the exercise is for you. In this exercise you simply walk up a step by putting your left foot in front of your right. Once both feet are on the step, step down and repeat for the exercise for 3 minutes.

This looks easy but when you use a 15-18 inch step it becomes a great cardio and leg conditioning exercise.

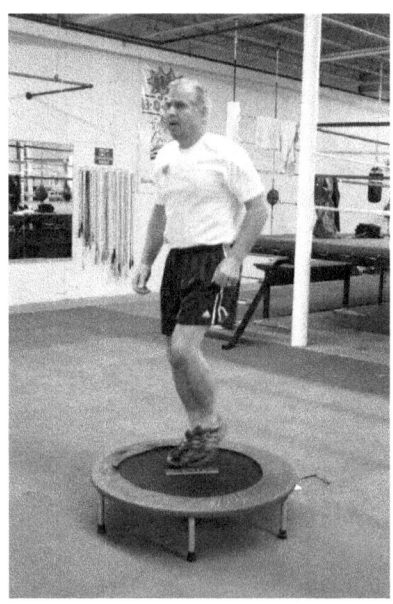

Rebounding

This is an incredible exercise. I purchased a mini-trampoline at Walmart for less than $30. Research has led some scientists to believe that jumping on a mini-trampoline is possibly the most effective exercise yet devised by man, especially because of the effect rebounding has on the lymph system in the body.

Squat Jump

To execute the squat jump stand with your feet square, a shoulder width apart. Squat down into the full squat position. As you stand up and reach your original standing position jump into the air.

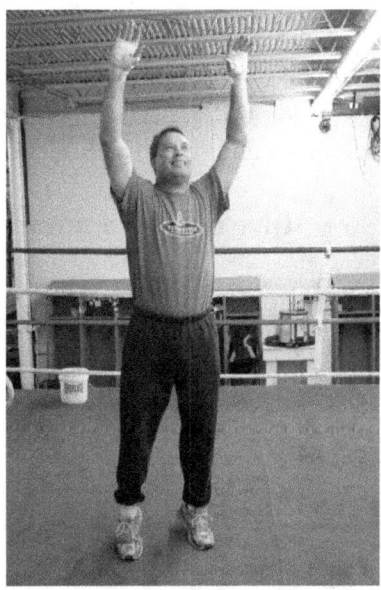

Squat jump

Dive Bombers

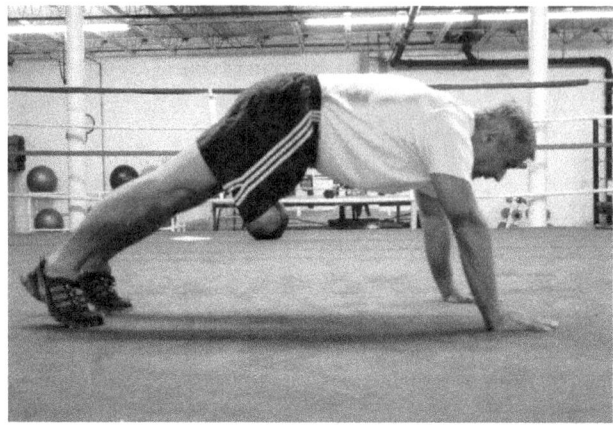

Start in the upright push-up position. Dive down and pretend you are crawling underneath a six inch rope. Fully extend your arms and arch your back. Now reverse the motion. This is a great cool down exercise for the back arms and legs. Do 3 sets of 10.

Dive Bomber Finish

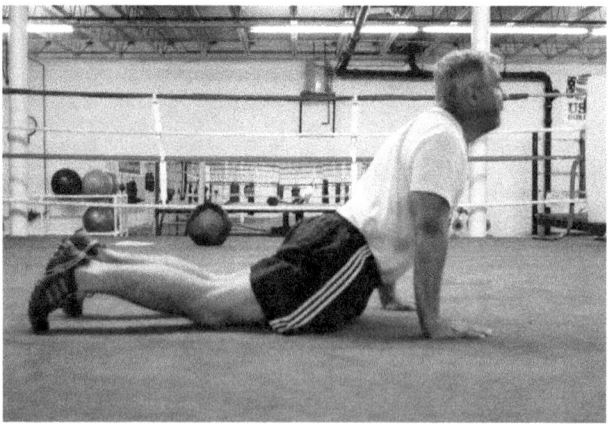

Dips

This is a great chest, shoulder, and triceps exercise. You can do this for three minutes you don't need help from anybody. Do 3 sets of 10 reps every other day with this exercise.

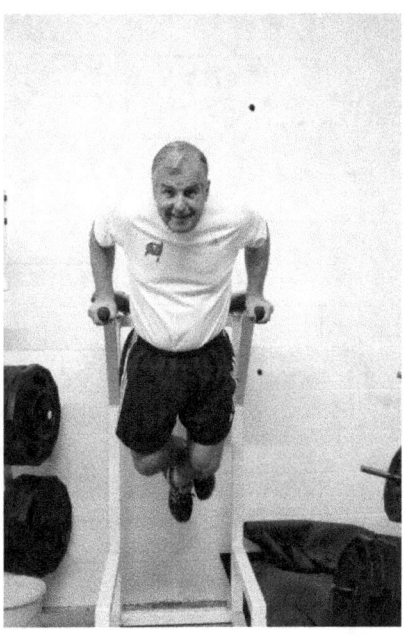

Close hand push-ups

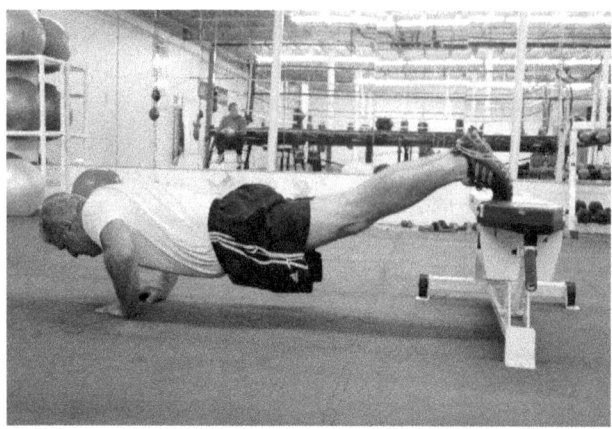

You may do the standard push-ups or increase the level of difficulty by doing them with both hands close together. For shaping and building the body, I recommend multiple sets of body shaping exercises.

Bench Dips

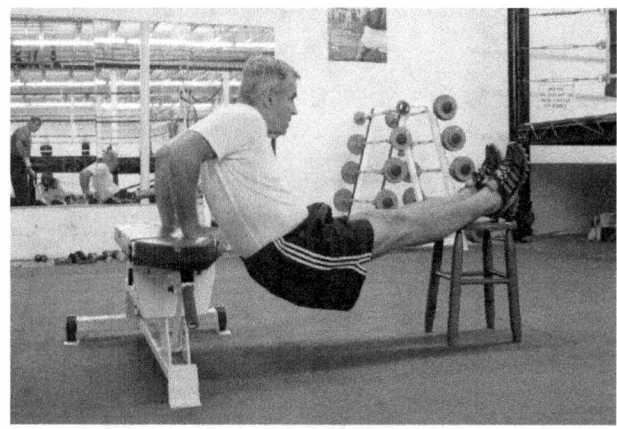

Bench dips is another great triceps exercise. 3 sets of 10 reps is good.

Hand stand push-ups

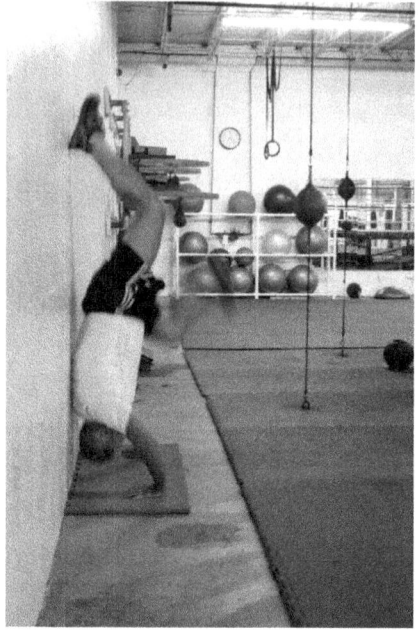

For athletes and those in really good condition this is a fun exercise.
Be very careful as it is fairly difficult.

Chin-ups

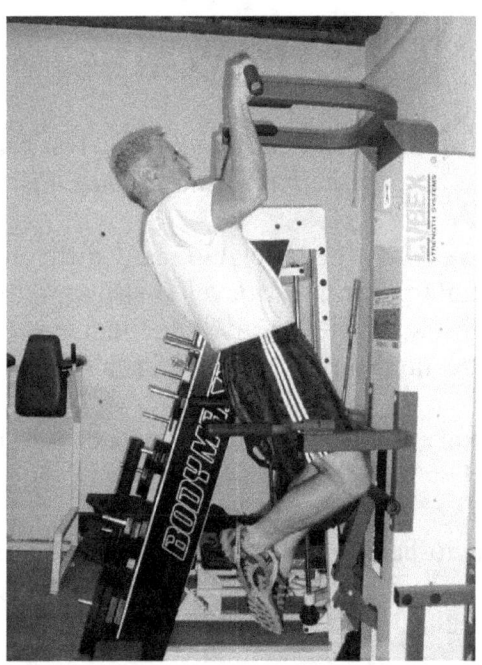

This is a great body building exercise for the upper-back (specifically the lats) and biceps. Don't feel bad if you can't do many reps at first. When I started training several months ago after a long lay-off I could only do 3 or 4 reps. Take your time with all of the exercises and slowly build your strength and endurance.

ROUND 12

AB WORK

"If you ever dreamed you could whip me, you better wake up and apologize." Muhammad Ali

Having a strong core is beneficial in many different areas. First of all if you are a fighter you must develop strong muscles that surround you're your ribs, solar plexus, liver and kidneys. One shot to an out of shape mid-section can end the fight instantly.

It's not necessary to have six pack abs because abdominal muscles can be bruised by an opponent's punches.

It doesn't hurt to have a little padding over your abs and your vital organs. But the mid section should be hard and tight to protect you from body punches.

When Ken Atkin was an amateur boxer, he fought several fights at heavyweight even though he was only about five feet, seven inches, tall. One night he was matched against James Gaines, a boxer who became a fringe heavyweight contender as a pro. As an amateur, Gaines was six feet, six inches tall and weighed at least 270 pounds and he had a huge "belly".

During the fight Atkin began to punch Gaines in his extremely large mid-section as hard as he could without doing any damage. Suddenly somebody from the crowd yelled and said - ***"You can hit that belly for a week and not hit the same spot."***

Fighters who are lean are almost always better boxers than fighters who are fat. However a little padding around the mid section that is tight will help protect your body.

In addition to protecting your body, having a strong mid-section will increase your power, speed and endurance.

Since having a strong core is critical for boxers and all other athletes as well, I've added a significant number of different abdominal exercises in this chapter to help you tighten up your mid-section.

Leg Throws

Start in the position illustrated in the photo below. Your workout partner will attempt to throw your legs to the floor while you resist. The finish position is in the second photo.

Leg throws start position

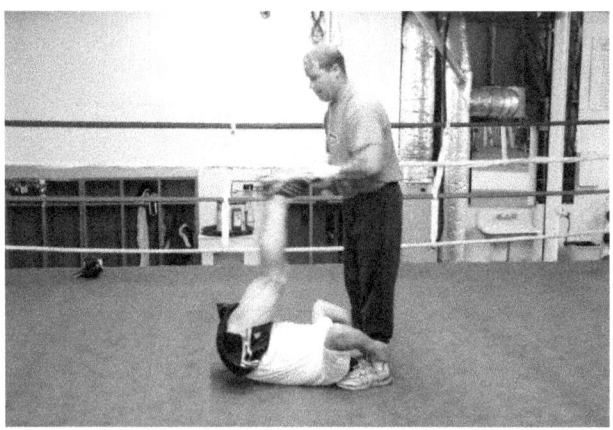

Leg throws finish position

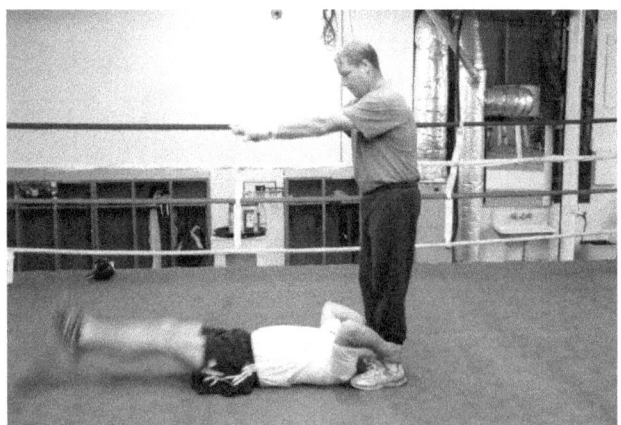

Glute Bridge

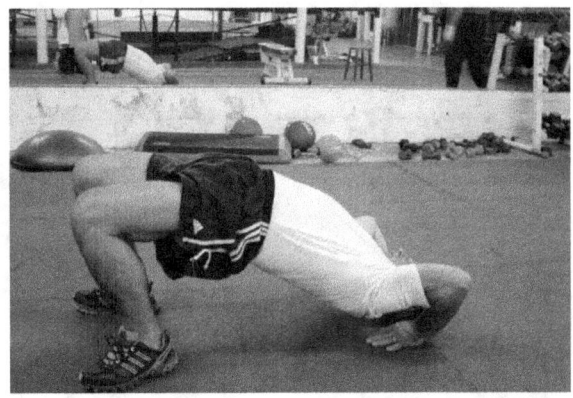

Start this exercise by lying on your back with your hands reversed and tucked under your shoulders. Arch your back into the upright position and return to your original position. This exercise is great for the lower back and your butt. If you can do 10 reps then that is excellent.

Ab-wheel

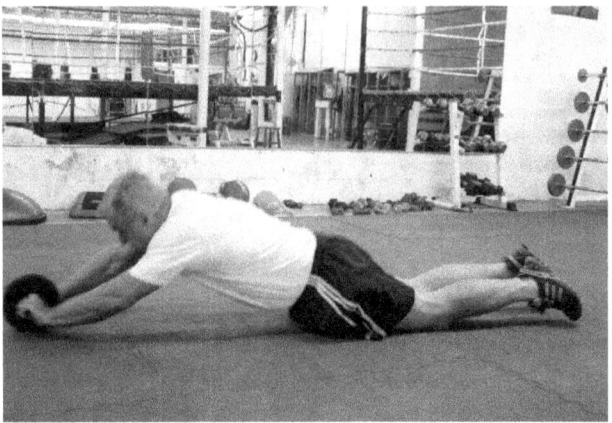

Start this exercise on your knees with the ab-wheel positioned in front of your body. Gently roll out until your body is parallel to the floor. If you've never done this exercise before, start very slowly with it if you want to be able to stand erect tomorrow. This is an incredible exercise for your mid-section. Although I've built up to 35 reps with this exercise I started by doing two or three reps at a time.

Sit-ups

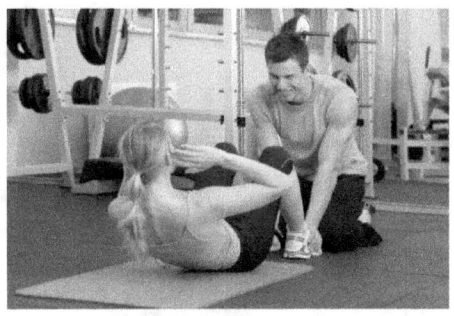

Need I say more?

Leg Raises

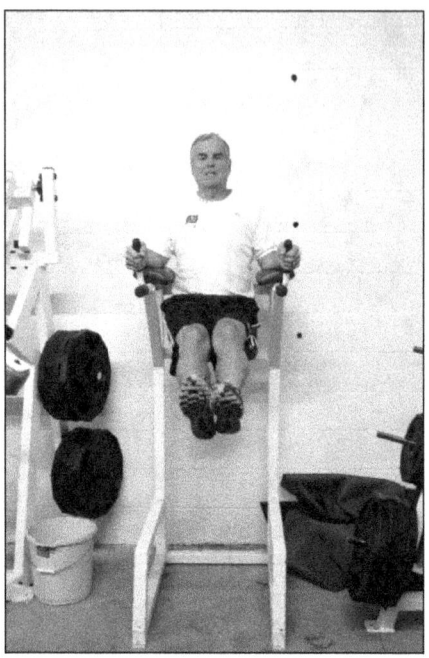

This is a variation of the hanging leg-raise exercise. This is an excellent exercise for lower abs. You can also do a similar leg raises by lying flat on a straight bench and raising your legs in the air and stopping them before they hit the floor as you lower them.

Around the world torso work

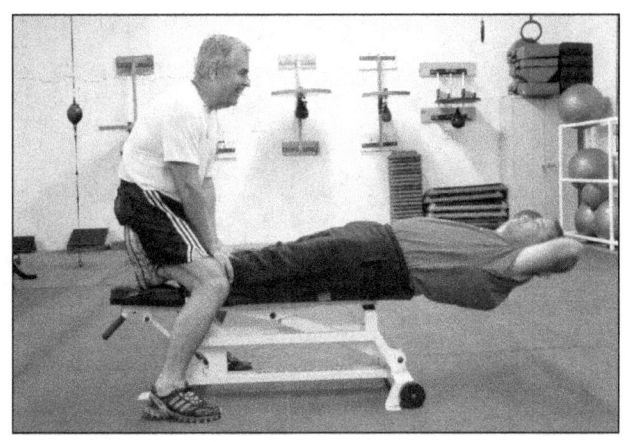

2nd position - do front, back, and both sides

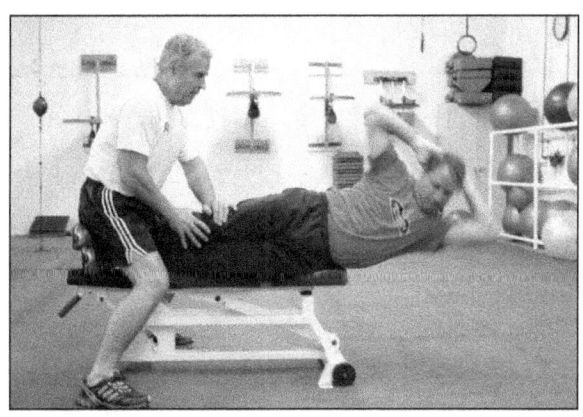

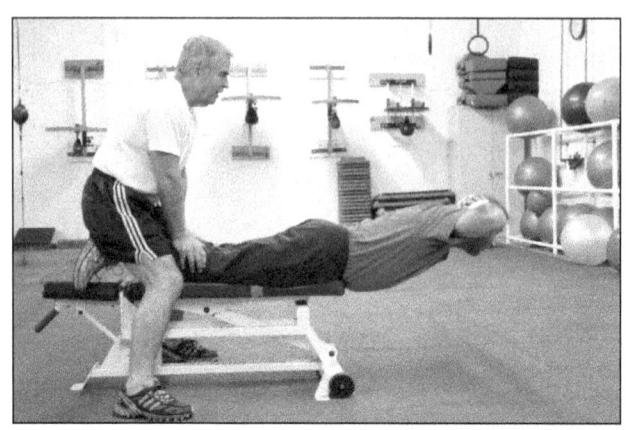

4th position

Ab work with medicine ball

In the following exercises the medicine ball is slammed into the abdomen of your partner while he flexes his abs. It is much easier than it looks.

Medicine ball ab-work

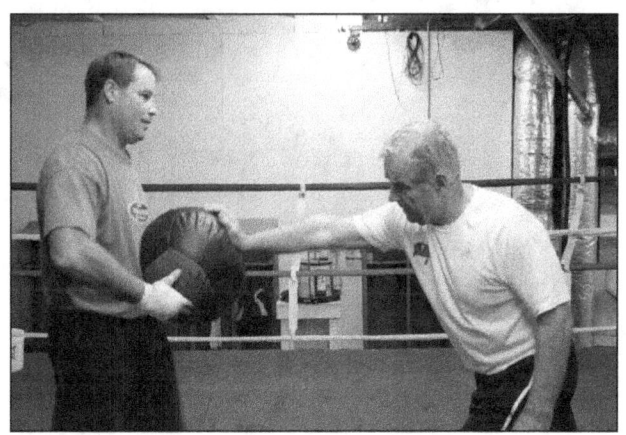

To the side

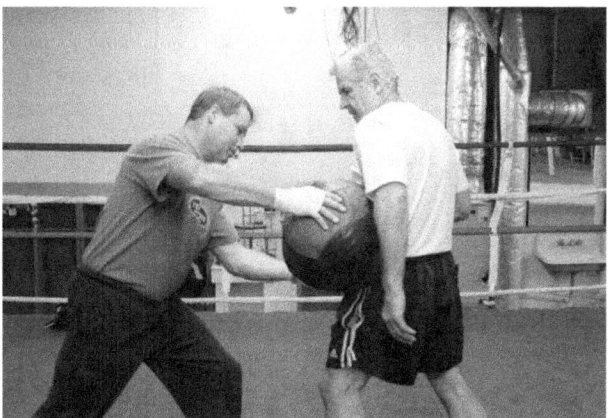

From above

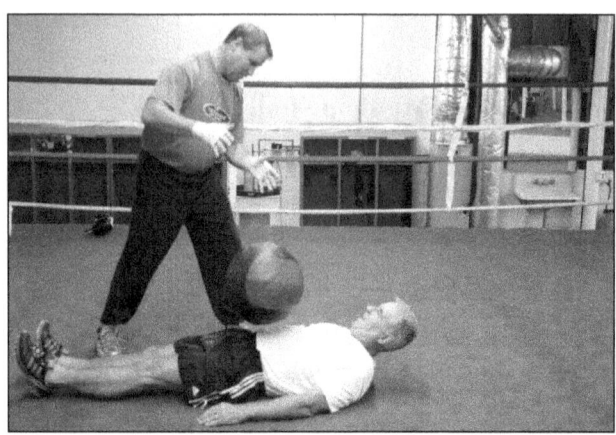

Road work

In addition to gym work, boxers also do road work. If you get a good gym workout three or four times a week and do your roadwork, running 2-3 miles three times a week, you will certainly improve your physical condition.

I would love to be your personal trainer. Unfortunately, I can't work with everyone individually. However we have filmed much of what I've taught to hundreds of other athletes over the years and it is available for you at www.ProBoxingTrainer.com

"I'm so fast I can turn the light off and be in bed before it's dark."
-Muhammad Ali

"Sports is the toy department of human life." -Howard Cosell

"The possession of muscular strength and the courage to use it in contests with other men for physical supremacy does not necessarily imply a lack of appreciation for the fine things in life."
-Jack Johnson

"The time may have come to say goodbye to Muhammad Ali, because very honestly, I don't think he can beat George Foreman."
-Howard Cosell

"Many people fail not so much because of their mistakes; they fail because they are afraid to try." -George Foreman

The Last Round

Making Weight

"If the money's right, I'm happy to bust up the other side of his face…No problem." -Lennox Lewis

In this chapter I want to give 7 helpful hints on losing fat and making weight.

1. Start by eliminating as much sugar, refined grains, and high sugar fruit from your diet as you can. Refined sugar, fruit sugar, and grain products when consumed cause a spike of insulin in your body.

   Insulin is referred to as the fat storage hormone because it converts carbohydrates into fat. Here's the "Real Deal" when you eat sugar, refined grain products, or high sugar fruit - your body quickly releases insulin, which in turn stores fat and also raises your cholesterol.

   If you need to lose weight you must eliminate white potatoes, corn, white rice, bread from refined flour, beets, carrots, refined sugar, corn syrup, molasses, honey, colas, and beer.
   All forms of sugar put your body into Fat Storage Mode!

2. Eliminate high - glycemic foods from your diet and eat only low - glycemic carbohydrates.

   The glycemic index (GI) is a numerical system of measuring how fast a carbohydrate triggers a rise in your blood sugar. The higher the number, the faster the rise in your blood sugar. Sugar, and refined carbohydrates like the ones mentioned above, cause a rapid elevation of your blood sugar. A low - glycemic food will not cause any significant spike and they will not add fat to your body. Protein and fat do not cause a rapid rise in blood sugar, only high sugar carbohydrates do.

- Low - glycemic carbohydrates are 55 or less on the Glycemic Index
- Medium-glycemic foods are 55-69
- High glycemic foods are 70 and above

Classification	GI range	Examples
Low GI	55 or less	most fruits and vegetables; legumes; some whole, intact grains; nuts; kidney beans; beets; chickpeas
Medium GI	56-69	whole wheat products, pita bread, basmati rice, grapes, sucrose, raisins, pumpernickel bread, cranberry juice, regular ice cream
High GI	70 and above	white bread, most white rices, corn flakes, extruded breakfast cereals, glucose, maltose, maltodextrins, white potato, pretzels

3. Drink lots of pure water. In order to burn calories you need to drink a lot of clean, fresh, alkaline, water daily. Being dehydrated not only slows down the fat burning process it also makes you weak and lethargic. The process of burning calories creates toxins or cause oxidation (think of the exhaust coming out of your car). Whenever we consume food, our bodies produce acid waste products such as carbon dioxide, lactic acid (that's where those sore muscles come form), and free radicals. Water plays a vital role in flushing these acidic poisons out of your body

4. When we consume mostly acidic foods and beverages, our bodies can become acidic. Acid based foods not only cause us to gain weight they can make us sick as well.

   Whenever we consume harmful acid food our own bodies create fat cells to store the acid. Cola drinks and other beverages are nearly as acidic as battery acid. If these acids weren't stored in fat cells they would be very detrimental to our health. Additionally our fat cells are reluctant to release fat when our body is acidic.

   Your stomach needs to be acidic to digest food but your bodily fluids need to be slightly alkaline to be healthy. Acidic foods are cooked and processed items. Alkaline foods are most fruits and vegetables. Start consuming more alkaline foods than acidic foods. When the body is alkaline the fat will melt off in record time.

5. If you are trying to make weight or just to lose weight so that you look better and are healthier, don't drink calories. Cola drinks, milk, and juice all have a significant number of calories and it is very easy to consume an extra 500 to 1000 calories per day by drinking caloric beverages. And some of the coffee beverages have 1500-2000 calories.

   It is so simple to exchange water or water with lemon in it instead of drinking high calorie beverages.

   I'm not trying to get you to give up everything you love forever, I'm just sharing some very healthy ways for you to drop fat and unwanted pounds.

6. If you want to make weight, lose fat, pounds, and or inches do not go hungry. It's actually much better to consume five small meals per day than it is to consume three larger meals.

At the beginning of each day prepare five small meals of about 300-325 calories each and eat every two hours during the day. This will keep your blood sugar stabilized and you have ravenous cravings. Always carry a healthy snack with you in case you do get hungry.

7. Exercise. If you are training in the sport of boxing you've definitely got the exercise part covered. There's nothing else for me to say about that.

I want to thank you for reading my book. And I want you to know that you can become a good boxer by applying the principles written in this book.

Feel free to contact me via email with any questions you may have.

ABOUT THE AUTHOR

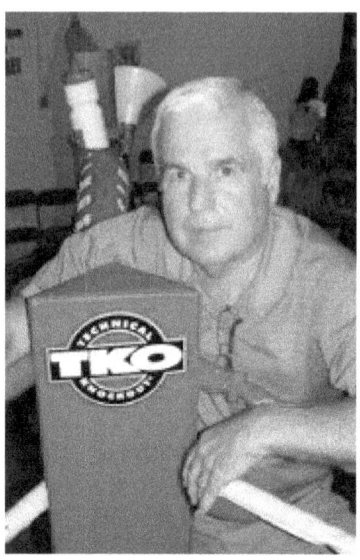

Kerry Pharr, is a fitness specialist, the host of the nationally broadcasted television program, *In Your Corner* and a former professional boxing trainer.

Pharr, served six years on the Tennessee Boxing Advisory Board. He owned and operated the renown Club Knockout Gym for over 20 years. Pharr is the author of three previous books including the health and fitness journal - *Young Again, How I Reversed the Aging Process, Restored my Health*, and *Lost Forty Pounds*. Over 400,000 people have benefited from his online video training programs.

www.ingramcontent.com/pod-product-compliance
Lightning Source LLC
Chambersburg PA
CBHW072336290526
45794CB00002B/894